Alive Natural Health Guides

Chia

USING THE ANCIENT SUPERFOOD

Beverly Lynn Bennett

Summertown
TENNESSEE

CONTENTS

& RECIPES

ACKNOWLEDGMENTS

I'd like to thank several people for their loving support and assistance during the writing of this book: Cynthia and Bob Holzapfel for their commitment to producing and publishing so many wonderful vegan and vegetarian lifestyle books and cookbooks, and for allowing me the opportunity to be a part of their respected family of authors. Jo Stepaniak, my friend and talented editor on this project, for her guidance and encouragement from the very beginning to the completion of this book. My husband, Ray Sammartano, for his love, support, and insightful comments, and more important, for being my chief taste tester during the recipe-development process. Luna, my feline companion, for supervising me in the kitchen while I was creating the recipes, and for the many purring sessions and snuggling lovefests on my lap while I sat at the computer. And last, all the vegans in the world for choosing to improve their lives, the lives of animals, and the future of this planet. Thank you for living with awareness and making a difference.

chia
A NUTRITIONAL POWERHOUSE

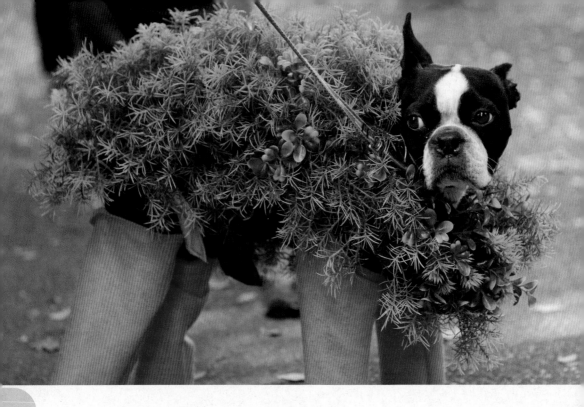

THE LEGENDARY CHIA SEED

We've all seen them on TV and in our local stores: those cute clay figurines with the green sprout-covered tops known as Chia Pets. Since their introduction in the 1980s, these little indoor topiaries have contributed greatly to renewed interest in chia seeds as a food source and cash crop. One of the latest crazes to hit the food scene, chia seeds might be new to you, but they've been cultivated and consumed for centuries—and rightfully so, as the chia seed is one petite powerhouse!

In the pages ahead, you'll find information about the many nutritional and health-promoting benefits of working chia seeds into daily meals. Plus, this book also presents more than twenty-five tasty recipes, all of which incorporate chia in one form or another. These recipes contain only vegan ingredients, and many are also gluten-free or include substitution suggestions. So get ready to look and feel like a super-new you, simply by eating this superfood—chia seeds!

What Are Chia Seeds?

Chia seeds (pronounced CHEE-ah) are harvested from the *Salvia hispanica* plant, which is a member of the mint family. This staple crop has been grown for centuries in North, Central, and South America. A single chia seed is tiny, much smaller in size than the average sesame, flax, or hemp seed. Chia seeds have a mild, slightly nutty flavor, and come in shades of speckled black and white.

White chia seeds are rarer than the black variety and as a result are more expensive. Although the type of soil in which chia seeds are grown can affect the seeds' nutritional content, most experts agree that there really isn't a significant nutritional difference between the white and black chia seeds.

Chia seeds are considered to be a whole food, as their bran, germ, and endosperm are still intact when they are packaged for sale. They are also mucilaginous, which means that when chia seeds get wet, they swell and secrete a sticky, gel-like substance. In turn, eating these seeds imparts a sense of fullness, which can help those who consume them to eat less and lose weight. Amazingly, chia seeds are capable of absorbing more than nine times their volume in liquid. The FDA classifies chia seeds as a food, not a supplement; therefore, they can be consumed without restrictions. Some experts even recommend feeding them to cats, dogs, and other animals.

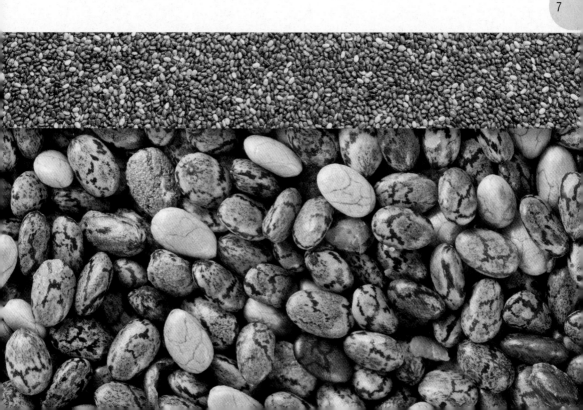

Early Chia Seed Cultivation and Uses

There is documented evidence that chia seeds were cultivated as early as 3500 BC. The tiny chia seeds were highly prized by many early civilizations of the Americas, including the ancient Aztecs and Mayans of what is now Mexico, who used them in many different ways. In fact, the word *chia* is derived from the Nahuatl (Aztec) word for "strength." The name of the Mexican state of Chiapas is derived from the word *chiapan*, meaning "river of chia"; it was named as such because it lies within the ancient Mayan territorial borders. Some historians believe that Aztec warriors and athletes could easily endure high levels of physical activity, long battles, and extensive journeys, maintaining their strength and stamina simply by consuming some water and a handful of chia seeds every few hours. That's truly incredible!

For sustenance, these ancient tribes would mix chia seeds with water to make a beverage. They also ate the seeds alone or mixed them with their other main crops of amaranth, beans, corn, and squash. The ground seeds were used to make a mush or porridge.

The tribes added chia seeds to their medicines and used them to seal wounds and prevent infections. They also pressed the tiny seeds between rocks to extract their oil for use in making body paints. The Aztecs and Mayans held chia in such esteem that their high priests even made offerings of the seeds to the gods during their religious rituals.

So why did chia seeds slip into obscurity and remain virtually unknown to most of the world? European explorers and rulers might have contributed to chia's fall from grace as a food source. In particular, as part of the Spanish conquest of the Americas, the invading Spaniards prohibited the so-called primitive and pagan religious rituals of the indigenous people, which often included the use of chia seeds. In an effort to weaken these tribes, the Spanish conquerors also banned the growing of many of their main crops, chia among them, and even went so far as to burn their agricultural fields. The Europeans feared that chia seeds and their properties of enhancing endurance and performance would make it impossible to control the native people and their precious territories.

Fortunately for us, the chia seed endured and continued to grow wild across much of the southwestern United States, Mexico, and Central America, and the indigenous people of these areas continued to consume chia seeds as part of their daily diet. Likewise, in the past few decades, chia seeds have been rediscovered by the masses, and we have agricultural and medical experts, in addition to health food advocates, to thank for the resurgence of interest in chia seeds and their consumption. Chia seeds are now being cultivated throughout the world, and as a result, these diminutive seeds have become a popular superfood and add-in ingredient in many food products. And it's quite possible that those infectious Chia Pet commercials have added to the name recognition and widespread acceptance as well.

Nutritional Benefits of Chia Seeds

The increased availability of chia seeds certainly has contributed greatly to renewed interest in them. However, the wide variety of nutritional benefits they provide is what has made them so popular with medical experts, nutritionists, athletes, raw foodists, and people trying to make health-promoting lifestyle changes. Naturally, the exact health benefits of chia seeds will vary slightly from person to person. Factors that could affect the health benefits obtained from chia seeds include any current or serious medical conditions, amount of exercise and physical activity engaged in, and the amount of chia seeds regularly consumed. Here are just a few of the reported benefits:

- decreased inflammation and joint pain
- lowered cholesterol levels
- increased energy levels
- enhanced athletic performance
- improved digestion and regularity
- augmented weight loss
- refined appearance of skin, hair, and nails

Even though they may be tiny, chia seeds are extremely nutritious. According to the United States Department of Agriculture (USDA), a 1-ounce serving (approximately 2 tablespoons) of chia seeds contains 137 calories, 11 grams of dietary fiber, 4 grams of protein, 9 grams of fat (1 gram of saturated fat), and 4 grams of omega-3 fatty acids. The following are some of the vitamins and minerals found in significant amounts in chia seeds: niacin, folic acid, calcium, magnesium, potassium, and iron; in lesser amounts are vitamins A, C, and E, and selenium. Adding chia seeds to your daily diet will also provide you with many beneficial antioxidants, which will help your body neutralize free radicals that can damage cells and cause oxidative stress, a condition that has been linked to degenerative diseases, such as Alzheimer's disease, cancer, cardiovascular disease, cataracts, cognitive impairment, immune dysfunction, macular degeneration, and Parkinson's disease.

Chia seeds are an excellent source of low-fat, plant-based protein and contain even more protein than wheat. Vegans and vegetarians will be glad to know that chia seeds, like soybeans, are considered to be a complete protein and contain all nine essential amino acids, which our bodies cannot manufacture and must be obtained through dietary sources.

Dietary fiber, found only in plant-based foods, is plentiful in chia seeds. It's important to eat adequate amounts of foods rich in both soluble and insoluble fiber for proper digestive and bowel health. Doing so can also help maintain proper weight, lower blood cholesterol levels, and reduce the risk of cardiovascular disease and some forms of cancer. Fortunately, chia seeds contain both types of fiber.

We also need to make sure that the foods we eat provide us with healthy sources of fat, or as medical professionals refer to them, essential fatty acids, also called EFAs. The two types are linoleic acid, also known as LA or omega-6 fatty acid, and alpha-linolenic acid, also known as ALA or omega-3 fatty acid. EFAs also must be obtained through food sources, and they are further converted by the body into other compounds needed to perform various physical and mental functions. Chia seeds are reputed to be the richest plant-based source of omega-3 fatty acids. Many people believe that seafood is the optimal dietary source of omega-3 fatty acids, but chia seeds can literally blow that notion out of the water, as gram for gram, chia seeds contain eight times the amount found in both wild and farmed salmon. Eating foods with high levels of omega-3 fatty acids has been shown to reduce inflammation, improve mental functions, and decrease the risk of chronic diseases, such as cancer, heart disease, and arthritis.

According to data from the USDA and several independent lab tests, a gram-to-gram comparison between some commonly consumed foods and chia seeds showed that 100 grams of chia seeds contain the following:

- 15 times the amount of magnesium as broccoli
- 9 times the amount of phosphorus and 5 times the amount of calcium as whole cow's milk
- 3 times the amount of protein as canned kidney beans
- 3 times the amount of iron as spinach
- 2 times the amount of selenium as flaxseeds
- 2 times the amount of potassium as bananas
- 2 times the amount of dietary fiber as bran flakes cereal

People concerned about heart disease will be pleased to know that chia seeds are free of cholesterol and trans fats and low in calories and sodium. And if you're among the ranks of thousands of people who suffer from

Nutritional value of 100 grams of chia compared to single servings of other foods

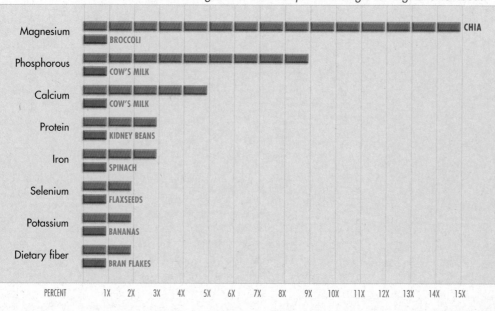

celiac disease or who are trying to limit their consumption of gluten-containing grains and by-products, you'll be happy to learn that chia seeds are gluten-free too.

Using Chia Seeds in Your Culinary Creations

Now that you know a little bit more about the various nutritional benefits that chia seeds have to offer, you're probably eager to get your hands on some and start working them into your daily meals more often. Luckily, chia seeds are now sold in most grocery and natural food stores and through online sources. I recommend buying organic chia seeds to avoid any agricultural contaminants. Whether to purchase black or white chia seeds depends on your preference; either variety can be used to make the recipes in this book.

Chia seeds are virtually tasteless, so you can easily use them to add a nutrient boost to daily meals. They are also easily digestible, and unlike flaxseeds, they don't need to be ground first before consumption. Thanks to a high antioxidant content, the oil in chia seeds will not become rancid if stored at room temperature or in direct sunlight, unlike the oils found in flax and other types of seeds and nuts. Store chia seeds in an airtight container in a cool, dry place; they will keep for about two years from the date of purchase.

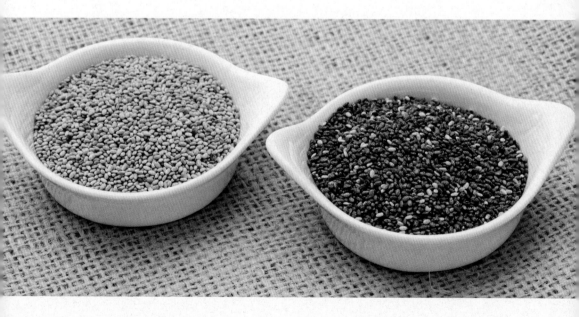

You'll be amazed how easy it can be to work chia seeds into your daily diet. You can eat them whole by the handful, stir them into juices or other beverages, or blend them into smoothies. Sprinkle them over your morning bowl of cereal or oatmeal, or scatter them atop cooked grains, noodle dishes, and other foods.

Chia seeds are easy to sprout (see page 28). As with other seeds, sprouting increases the seed's nutritional content. Chia sprouts are a delicious addition to sandwiches and salads.

Whole chia seeds and chia seed gel (see page 16) can be used to thicken soups, stews, and sauces or to replace some or even all of the oil in salad dressings and other recipes. Chia seed gel can be used as a binder in veggie burgers and meatless loaves and as an egg replacer in baked goods and desserts. The whole seeds can also be ground into a fine flour or coarse meal for use in baked goods, veggie burgers, and other dishes.

These are just a few of the tasty ways to enjoy chia seeds; the recipes in this book provide more examples. I hope they will inspire you to use your own culinary creativity and to start adding chia seeds to all your recipes with abandon.

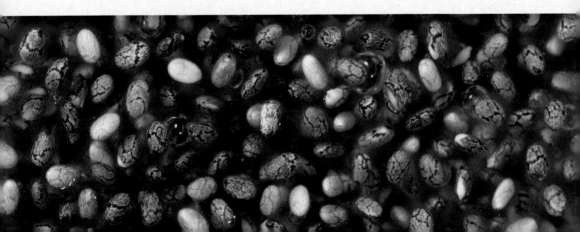

beverages and breakfast ideas

chia **Seed Gel**

YIELD: ¾ CUP

Simple to make, chia seed gel is virtually flavorless but can lend a tremendous boost of nutrition to whatever you add it to. This thick gel has an endless amount of uses and can work in recipes as a replacement for eggs, oil, or margarine. It can also act as a binder or thickener in baked goods, beverages, sauces, salad dressings, and soups, and can be used in both sweet and savory dishes. It's important to make chia seed gel using filtered water to avoid concentrating the harsh chemicals and compounds often found in tap water.

¾ cup **filtered water**

4 teaspoons **chia seeds**

Put the water and chia seeds in a small bowl and whisk until well combined. Set aside for 15 minutes to thicken. Whisk again to break up any clumps of chia seeds. Transfer to a glass jar with a tight-fitting lid or other airtight container. Stored in the refrigerator, Chia Seed Gel will keep for 2 weeks.

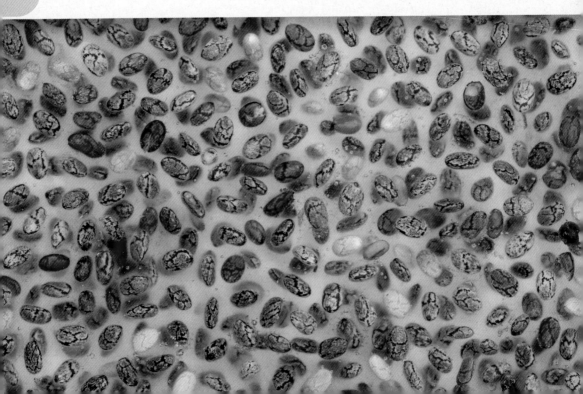

Chia *fresca*

Chia fresca, also known as *iskiate*, is a light and refreshing citrus-flavored drink made by many of the indigenous people of the southwestern United States and Mexico. This energizing beverage is a great way to kick-start your day and to keep you hydrated during exercise. Chia fresca is commonly made with either lemon or lime juice, but you can also use orange, satsuma, or grapefruit juice.

10 ounces **cold filtered water**

Juice of 1 large **lime** or ½ large **lemon** (2 to 3 tablespoons)

1 teaspoon **agave nectar** or other sweetener, plus more as needed

2 teaspoons **chia seeds**

Pour the water and lime juice into a large glass and whisk until well combined. Taste and add agave nectar as desired.

Whisk in the chia seeds and let thicken for 10 minutes. Before drinking, whisk the beverage again to break up any clumps of chia seeds.

TIP: For added flavor and visual appeal, garnish with a slice of lime or add half of the squeezed lime. If you like mint, garnish with a sprig of fresh mint or a few chopped mint leaves.

FRUITY CHIA FRESCA: Replace the water with fruit juice, such as raspberry, cherry, or pomegranate, or a fruit juice blend.

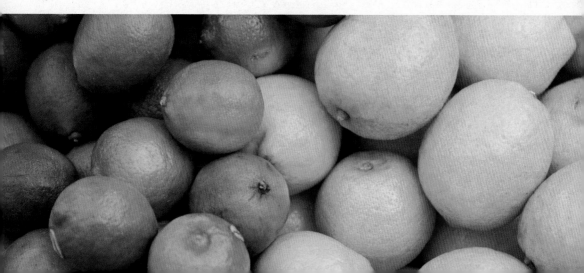

Paradise *smoothie*

YIELD: 2½ CUPS, 2 SERVINGS

Frosty and fruity, this island-inspired smoothie is the perfect way to start your day. It's made with a combination of banana, papaya, coconut water, macadamia nuts, dates, and omega-rich hemp and chia seeds.

1½ cups **coconut water**

⅓ cup **raw macadamia nuts**

2 tablespoons **hempseeds**

½ teaspoon **vanilla extract**

1 large **banana, broken into chunks**

1 cup **frozen papaya or mango chunks**

3 **pitted dates**

1½ tablespoons **chia seeds**

Put the coconut water, macadamia nuts, hempseeds, and vanilla extract in a blender and process until well combined. Add the banana, papaya, dates, and chia seeds and process until smooth. Serve immediately.

TIP: If you can't find frozen papaya chunks, use the same amount of fresh papaya and add ½ cup of ice cubes.

GREEN PARADISE SMOOTHIE: Add 2 cups of baby spinach or other leafy greens, stemmed and lightly packed.

HAWAIIAN ISLAND SMOOTHIE: Replace the coconut water with 1 (6-ounce) container of coconut yogurt and 1 cup of coconut milk beverage.

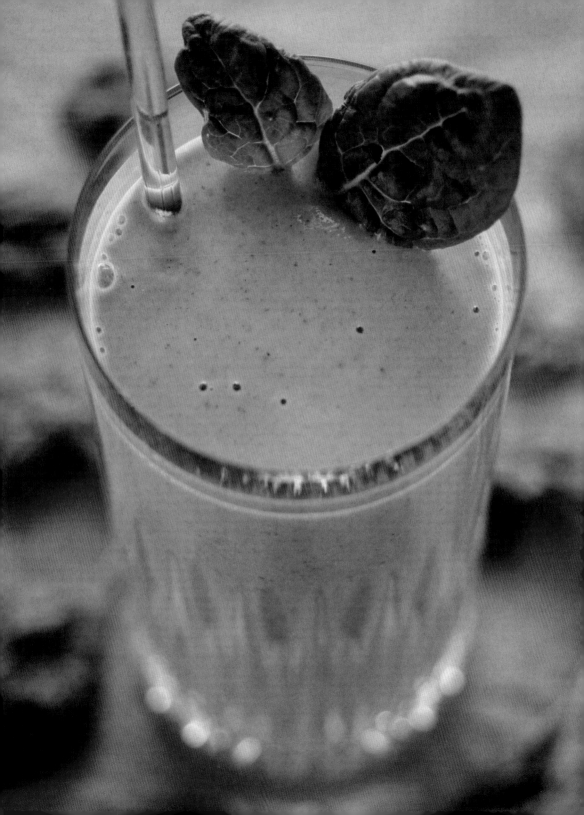

mishmash Hash

YIELD: 6 CUPS, 6 SERVINGS

Hash is a very forgiving dish to make because you can add or substitute almost any vegetables you like to it and it will still turn out delicious. And like many one-pot meals, it doesn't need a lot of babysitting. This version features chopped potatoes, kale, and aromatic vegetables. The final addition of sunflower, hemp, and chia seeds adds a crunchy counterbalance to the sautéed veggies.

4 **red-skinned potatoes**, scrubbed and cubed

1½ tablespoons **olive oil**

2 **carrots**, diced

1 cup diced **red or yellow onion**

1 **green or red bell pepper**, diced

1 large **stalk celery**, cut in half lengthwise and thinly sliced

1½ tablespoons minced **garlic**

2 teaspoons **Italian seasoning blend**

1 teaspoon **chili powder**

¾ teaspoon **smoked paprika**, or ¼ teaspoon **chipotle chili powder**

¾ teaspoon **sea salt or seasoned salt**

¼ teaspoon freshly **ground pepper**

3 cups **kale or other leafy greens**, stemmed and cut into very thin strips, packed

½ cup **frozen peas**

¼ cup chopped **fresh parsley**, lightly packed

2 tablespoons **nutritional yeast flakes**

¼ cup **chia seeds**

¼ cup **raw or roasted sunflower seeds**

2 tablespoons **hempseeds**

Put the potatoes and olive oil in a large cast-iron or nonstick skillet and cook over medium-high heat, stirring occasionally, for 5 minutes. Add the carrots, onion, bell pepper, and celery and cook, stirring occasionally, until starting to soften, about 5 minutes. Add the garlic, Italian seasoning blend, chili powder,

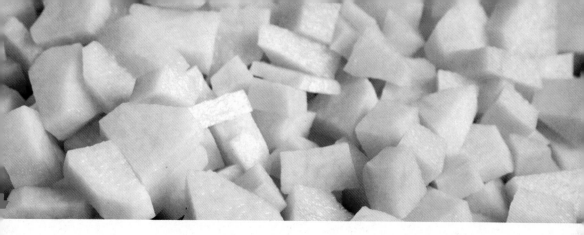

smoked paprika, salt, and pepper and cook, stirring occasionally, until well combined, about 1 minute.

Add the kale, peas, parsley, and nutritional yeast flakes and cook, stirring occasionally, until the kale has wilted and the other vegetables are tender, 3 to 5 minutes. Remove from the heat and stir in the chia seeds, sunflower seeds, and hempseeds. Serve hot.

VARIATION: Replace any of the suggested vegetables with others that you prefer, such as broccoli, cauliflower, green onions, shallots, sweet potatoes, turnips, or zucchini.

CHECKERED FLANNEL HASH: Replace 2 of the potatoes with 2 beets, peeled and cubed.

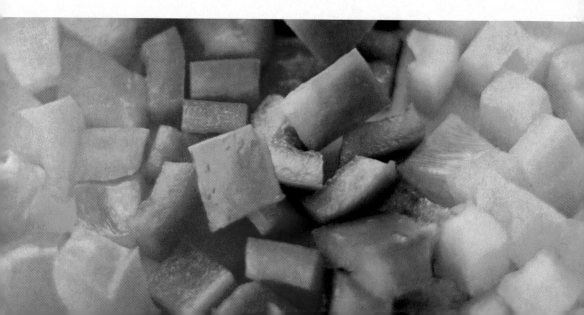

wholesome Waffle and Pancake Mix and Batter

Whether you're cooking for one or for a crowd, you can whip up a batch of waffles or pancakes in minutes and with minimal effort by keeping this dry ingredient mix on hand. Simply measure out the desired amount of mix, and by the time your griddle or waffle iron is hot, the nutrient-rich batter will be ready to go. Serve the pancakes or waffles with warm maple syrup or your favorite toppings.

WAFFLE AND PANCAKE MIX

1½ cups **whole wheat flour**

1½ cups **white whole wheat flour**

¾ cup ground **flaxseeds or flax-seed meal**

¼ cup **chia seeds**

¼ cup **coconut sugar or unbleached cane sugar**

2 tablespoons aluminum-free **baking powder**

2 teaspoons **ground cinnamon**

1 teaspoon **sea salt**

To make the mix, put the whole wheat flour, white whole wheat flour, flaxseeds, chia seeds, sugar, baking powder, cinnamon, and salt in a large bowl and whisk until well combined. Stored in an airtight container in the refrigerator or freezer, Wholesome Waffle and Pancake Mix will keep for 6 months.

To make pancake or waffle batter, pour the nondairy milk and vinegar into a small measuring cup or small bowl, stir until well combined, and let thicken for 5 minutes. Put the dry mix in a medium bowl. Add the thickened nondairy milk mixture, oil, and vanilla extract and whisk until just combined.

If making pancakes, lightly oil a large cast-iron or nonstick skillet, or a griddle, or mist it with cooking spray. Heat over medium heat. When the skillet is hot, pour the batter into it using ⅓ cup of batter for each pancake. Cook until the edges of the pancakes are slightly dry and bubbles appear on top, 2 to 3 minutes. Flip the pancakes over with a spatula and cook until golden brown on the other side, 2 to 3 minutes. Lightly oil the skillet again and repeat the cooking procedure with the remaining batter. Serve hot.

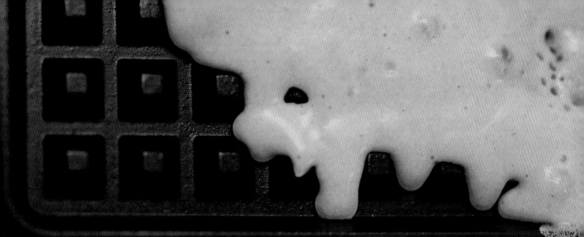

BATTER (MAKES 4 PANCAKES OR 3 WAFFLES)

¾ cup **nondairy milk**

1 teaspoon **cider vinegar or lemon juice**

1 cup (for pancakes) or 1¼ cups (for waffles) **Wholesome Waffle and Pancake Mix**

1 tablespoon **coconut oil, melted, or other oil**

1 teaspoon **vanilla extract**

If making waffles, preheat a waffle iron according to the manufacturer's instructions. When the waffle iron is hot, lightly oil it or mist it with cooking spray. Depending on the size of the waffle iron, ladle ¾ to 1 cup of batter onto the iron and cook according to the manufacturer's instructions or until golden brown. Lightly oil the waffle iron again and repeat the cooking procedure with the remaining batter. Serve hot.

TIP: Gently mix your favorite additions into the prepared batter, such as coarsely chopped nuts or seeds, coarsely chopped or sliced fruit, fresh or frozen berries, or chocolate or carob chips.

WHEAT-FREE WHOLESOME WAFFLE AND PANCAKE MIX: Replace both of the whole wheat flours with spelt flour or barley flour.

GLUTEN-FREE WHOLESOME WAFFLE AND PANCAKE MIX: Replace both of the whole wheat flours with buckwheat flour or a gluten-free baking blend.

Good Morning *muffins*

YIELD: 12 MUFFINS

Whole wheat pastry flour, rolled oats, and your fruit of choice boost the fiber content of these tasty muffins, while applesauce, ground flaxseeds, and chia seed gel play dual roles as replacements for both eggs and oil in the batter.

1 cup **soy milk or other nondairy milk**

1½ teaspoons **cider vinegar or lemon juice**

6 tablespoons **applesauce**

2 tablespoons **Chia Seed Gel** (page 16)

1½ teaspoons **vanilla extract**

1½ cups **whole wheat pastry flour**

½ cup **old-fashioned rolled oats**

½ cup **turbinado sugar, coconut sugar, or light brown sugar,** lightly packed

2 teaspoons **ground flaxseeds or flaxseed meal**

1½ teaspoons **aluminum-free baking powder**

1 teaspoon **ground cinnamon**

¾ teaspoon **baking soda**

¼ teaspoon **sea salt**

1 cup **fresh or unthawed frozen berries** (such as blueberries, raspberries, or strawberries) or coarsely chopped fruit (such as apples, bananas, cherries, or peaches)

Preheat the oven to 400 degrees F. Lightly oil 12 muffin cups or mist them with cooking spray. Alternatively, line them with paper liners or use silicone muffin cups.

Put the soy milk and vinegar in a measuring cup or small bowl and stir until well combined. Let thicken for 5 minutes. Add the applesauce, Chia Seed Gel, and vanilla extract to the thickened soy milk mixture and whisk until well combined.

Put the flour, oats, sugar, flaxseeds, baking powder, cinnamon, baking soda, and salt in a large bowl and whisk until well combined. Add the wet ingredients to the dry ingredients and stir until just combined. Gently stir in the fruit.

Fill the prepared muffin cups using a ¼-cup ice-cream scoop or until three-quarters full. Bake for 18 to 20 minutes, or until a toothpick inserted in the center of a muffin comes out clean. Allow the muffins to cool slightly in the pan and then transfer them to a rack to cool as desired. Serve warm or at room temperature. Stored in an airtight container or ziplock bag, Good Morning Muffins will keep for 3 days.

VARIATIONS: Replace one-third of the fruit with ⅓ cup of coarsely chopped nuts, seeds, or dried fruits (such as raisins or goji berries, or dried cranberries or cherries). To vary the flavor of the muffins, replace the applesauce with an equal amount of mashed banana, or pumpkin or winter squash purée.

GLUTEN-FREE GOOD MORNING MUFFINS: Replace the whole wheat pastry flour with an equal amount of gluten-free baking mix and add ¾ teaspoon of xanthan gum.

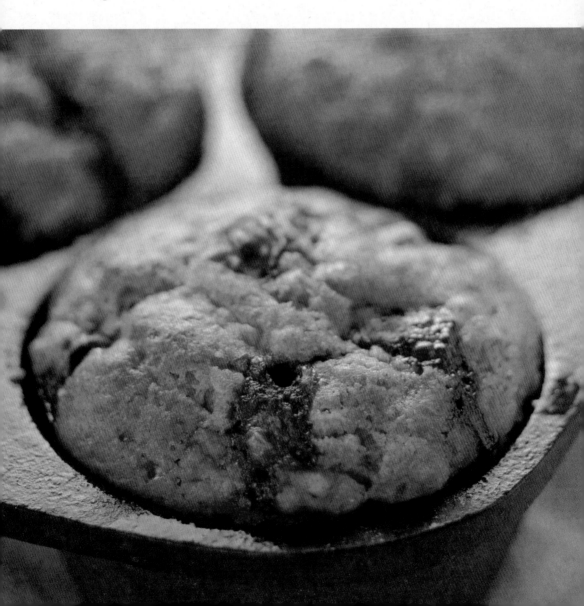

porridge with Chia Seeds, Nuts, and Fruit

YIELD: 2½ CUPS, 2 SERVINGS

Blending chia seeds with almonds, dates, and spices, and then chilling the mixture, magically transforms it into a thick and creamy concoction reminiscent of cooked grain-based porridge. Crisp apples, sweet raisins, and crunchy walnuts top the individual servings.

1½ cups **water**

½ cup **raw whole almonds**

4 **pitted dates**

1 teaspoon **vanilla extract**

½ teaspoon **ground cinnamon,** plus more for garnish

3 tablespoons **chia seeds**

1 **apple,** cored and chopped

¼ cup coarsely chopped **raw walnuts**

2 tablespoons **raisins**

Put the water, almonds, dates, vanilla extract, and cinnamon in a blender and process until smooth, about 1 minute. Scrape down the sides of the blender jar with a spatula. Add the chia seeds and process until smooth and well combined, about 15 seconds.

Transfer the mixture to a glass bowl with a tight-fitting lid or other airtight container and refrigerate for 8 to 12 hours to allow the flavors to blend and the mixture to thicken. Alternatively, if you're in a hurry, refrigerate the mixture for at least 30 minutes.

Before serving, stir the mixture to break up any clumps of chia seeds. Evenly divide the mixture between 2 bowls. Top each serving with half of the apple, 2 tablespoons of the walnuts, 1 tablespoon of the raisins, and a sprinkle of additional cinnamon. Serve immediately.

VARIATIONS: Substitute other varieties of fresh fruit, berries, nuts, or seeds to suit your taste and the seasonal availability of ingredients. Here are a few combination suggestions:

- 1 peach or nectarine, chopped, ¼ cup sliced almonds, and 1 tablespoon coarsely chopped crystallized ginger
- 1 mango, chopped, ¼ cup coarsely chopped raw macadamia nuts, 1 tablespoon unsweetened shredded dried coconut
- 3 dried apricots, coarsely chopped, ¼ cup pistachios, 2 tablespoons goji berries, and 2 tablespoons currants or dried cranberries

options for lunch

Chia Seed *sprouts*

You don't need a cute little figurine or even a handful of dirt to grow your own chia seed sprouts. With only a large dinner plate, a glass pie pan, and a spray bottle filled with water—plus a few days of diligence—you can grow a batch of fresh sprouts that you can toss into salads, add to sandwiches, or use any way you like.

1 tablespoon **chia seeds**

Water

Put the chia seeds on a large dinner plate. Gently move the plate to spread the chia seeds into a single layer.

Fill a clean spray bottle with water. Evenly spray a fine mist of water over the chia seeds. Place a glass pie pan upside down on top of the plate to cover (like a lid for a pot). Put the sprout setup on a counter or table away from direct sunlight or overhead lighting.

Twice a day, evenly spray a light mist of water over the chia seeds and cover the plate again with the pie pan. Continue this procedure until the chia seeds begin to have small green leaves and their stems are several inches long, 5 to 7 days. The sprouts are ready to harvest when they have very dark green leaves.

Put the sprouts in a fine-mesh strainer and gently rinse under running water to separate them. Allow the sprouts to drain thoroughly, and then transfer them to an airtight container. Stored in the refrigerator, Chia Seed Sprouts will keep for 3 days.

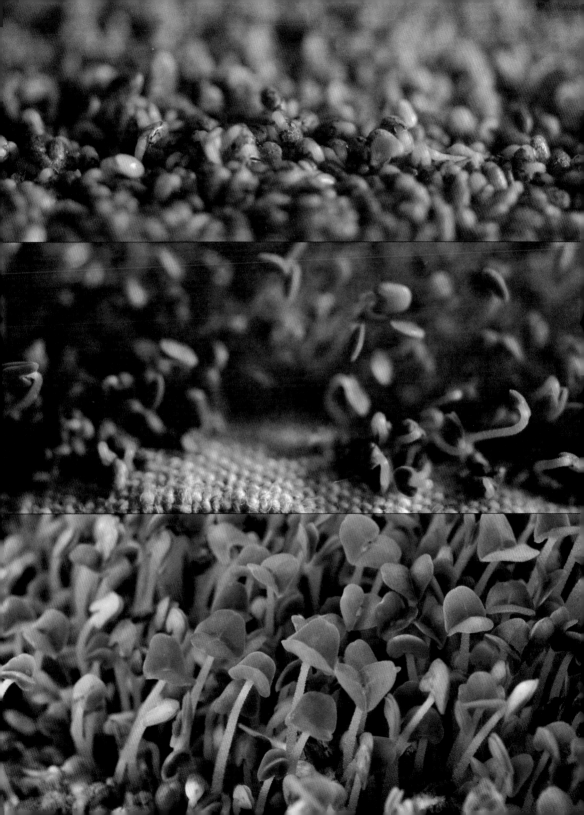

rainbow Veggie and Greens Salad with Cha-Cha Chia Seed Dressing

YIELD: 5 SERVINGS

Hearty and crisp, this salad features a vibrant blend of mixed greens and crunchy fresh veggies in most of the colors of the rainbow. Forget about adding oil to thicken the creamy and zesty Italian-style dressing, and instead use healthful chia seeds.

CHA-CHA CHIA SEED DRESSING (1 CUP)

⅔ cup **soy milk** or other nondairy milk

2 tablespoons **lemon juice**

2 tablespoons **plain vegan yogurt**

2 large **cloves garlic,** minced

2 teaspoons **nutritional yeast flakes**

1½ teaspoons **Italian seasoning blend,** or ½ teaspoon dried basil, ½ teaspoon dried oregano, and ½ teaspoon dried thyme

1½ teaspoons **onion powder**

¾ teaspoon **crushed red pepper flakes**

½ teaspoon **chia seeds**

½ teaspoon **spicy brown mustard** or Dijon mustard

¼ teaspoon **sea salt**

¼ teaspoon **freshly ground pepper**

To make the dressing, put all of the dressing ingredients in a blender and process until smooth, stopping once or twice to scrape down the sides of the blender jar. Transfer the dressing to an airtight container. Stored in the refrigerator, Cha-Cha Chia Seed Dressing will keep for 7 days.

SALAD (10 CUPS)

4 cups **mixed baby greens**

1 cup shredded **green cabbage or Savoy cabbage**

1 cup shredded **red cabbage**

1 cup shredded **carrot**

2 large stalks **celery**, thinly sliced

1 cup thinly sliced **cucumber** (quarter lengthwise before slicing)

½ cup halved and thinly sliced **radishes**

1 cup **Chia Seed Sprouts** (page 28)

To make the salad, put the baby greens, green cabbage, red cabbage, carrot, celery, cucumber, and radishes in a large bowl and gently toss. Scatter the sprouts over the top of the salad mixture. Drizzle the dressing over individual servings as desired.

TIPS: Make this salad with one or more other varieties of leafy greens, such as Swiss chard, green or purple kale, spinach, or arugula. For a wrap, roll up portions of this salad in a tortilla or stuff it into pita halves. You can also use Cha-Cha Chia Seed Dressing to top your favorite blend of mixed greens or veggie slaws, or to perk up pasta or grain-based salad combinations.

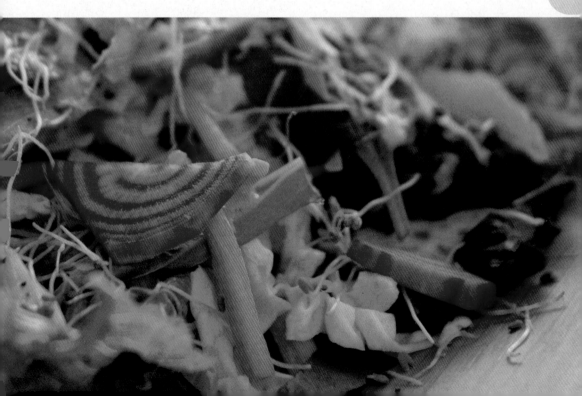

Fruit, Nut, and Seed Tofu *salad*

YIELD: 4 CUPS, 8 SERVINGS

Seasoned and baked cubes of tofu are the perfect stand-in for chicken, as are chia seeds for poppy seeds, in this updated and veganized version of poppy seed chicken salad; juicy grapes, dried cranberries, and sliced almonds enhance this pairing. Serve this tofu salad on a bed of lettuce or atop crackers or flatbread, or use it as a filling for sandwiches or wraps.

CHICKEN-STYLE TOFU

1 pound **firm or extra-firm regular tofu,** cut into 1-inch cubes or strips

2 tablespoons **reduced-sodium soy sauce**

1 tablespoon **toasted sesame oil or other oil**

1 teaspoon **onion powder**

1 teaspoon **garlic powder**

1½ tablespoons **nutritional yeast flakes**

To make the chicken-style tofu, preheat the oven to 400 degrees F. Line a large baking sheet with parchment paper or a silicone baking mat.

Put the tofu on the prepared baking sheet. Sprinkle with the soy sauce, sesame oil, onion powder, and garlic powder and toss well with your hands to evenly coat the tofu. Spread the tofu into a single layer and evenly sprinkle half of the nutritional yeast flakes over the top. Bake for 15 minutes.

Remove from the oven. Stir the tofu with a spatula and spread into a single layer again. Evenly sprinkle the remaining nutritional yeast flakes over the tofu. Bake for 10 to 15 minutes longer, until the tofu is golden brown and crisp around the edges. Let cool completely before making the salad.

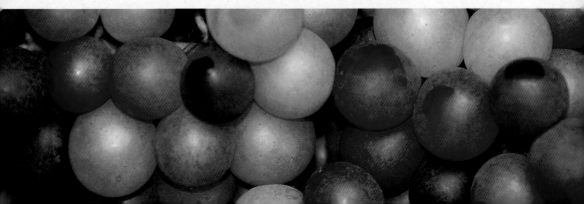

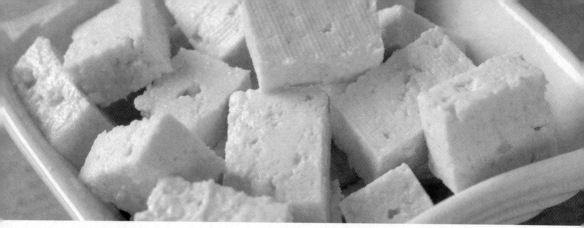

SALAD

½ cup halved **seedless green grapes**

½ cup halved **seedless red grapes**

1 large stalk **celery**, diced

½ cup **sliced almonds**

½ cup **dried cranberries**

¼ cup thinly sliced **green onion**

1 cup **vegan mayonnaise**

2 tablespoons **lemon juice**

1½ tablespoons **chia seeds**

1 teaspoon dried **dill weed**

Sea salt

Freshly ground **pepper**

To make the salad, put the tofu, green grapes, red grapes, celery, almonds, dried cranberries, and green onion in a large bowl and gently stir until well combined. Add the mayonnaise, lemon juice, chia seeds, and dill weed and gently stir until well combined. Season with salt and pepper to taste and gently stir again. Serve immediately or thoroughly chilled.

AUTUMN FRUIT, NUT, AND SEED TOFU SALAD: Replace the green grapes with 1 small apple, cored and diced, and replace the sliced almonds with ⅔ cup of coarsely chopped pecans.

Chia Veggie *burgers*

With the help of your food processor, these tasty bean- and veggie-based burgers come together in just minutes. Serve them on plates or burger buns with your favorite condiments and all the trimmings.

1 (15-ounce) can salt-free **white beans or chickpeas**, drained and rinsed

1 cup **kale or spinach**, stemmed and lightly packed

1 large stalk **celery**, cut into 4 pieces

1 large **carrot**, cut into 4 pieces

½ **red onion**, cut into 4 pieces

½ **red bell pepper**, seeded and cut into 4 pieces

¼ cup fresh **parsley**, lightly packed

2 tablespoons **spicy brown mustard or Dijon mustard**

2 tablespoons **nutritional yeast flakes**

1½ teaspoons **chili powder**

1½ teaspoons **dried thyme**

1½ teaspoons **garlic powder**

1½ teaspoons **ground cumin**

1½ teaspoons **smoked paprika**

½ teaspoon **sea salt**

¼ teaspoon **freshly ground pepper**

⅓ cup **raw or roasted sunflower seeds**

2 tablespoons **chia seeds**

2 tablespoons **hempseeds**

1 cup **chickpea flour, whole wheat flour, or other flour**

Put the beans, kale, celery, carrot, red onion, red bell pepper, parsley, mustard, nutritional yeast flakes, chili powder, thyme, garlic powder, cumin, smoked paprika, salt, and pepper in a food processor and process until coarsely ground, stopping occasionally to scrape down the sides of the container with a rubber spatula.

Transfer the bean mixture to a medium bowl. Add the sunflower seeds, chia seeds, and hempseeds and stir until well combined. Add the chickpea flour and stir until well combined.

Line a large baking sheet with parchment paper or a silicone baking mat. Using ½ cup measuring cup, prepare each patty by lightly filling and gently packing the burger mixture into the cup with the back of a spoon. Flip the measuring cup over onto the prepared baking sheet and tap the cup to release the bean mixture. Flatten each portion into a patty. Refrigerate the patties for at least 1 hour to let them firm up slightly.

Preheat the oven to 375 degrees F. Bake the patties for 15 minutes, until golden brown on top. Flip the patties over with a spatula and bake for 10 to 15 minutes longer, until the burgers are golden brown on both sides.

TIPS: If you prefer, the burgers can be cooked in an oiled skillet on the stove top over medium-high heat until golden brown on both sides. Baked or fried burgers can be stored in an airtight container in the freezer for up to 3 months. Reheat the frozen patties in a 350 degree F oven or in a skillet over medium heat until hot, about 15 minutes.

INDIAN-STYLE CHIA VEGGIE BURGERS: Prepare the recipe using chickpeas, omit the chili powder and smoked paprika, and add 1 tablespoon of curry powder or garam masala.

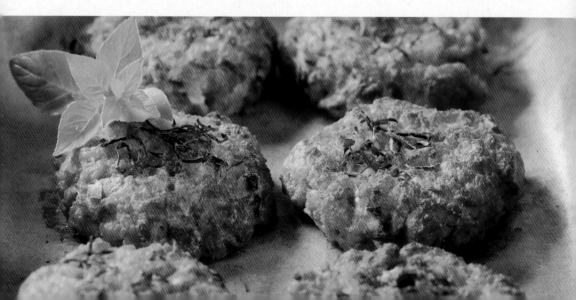

california **Club Sandwiches**

These veggie-centric club sandwiches consist of stacked layers of colorful and crisp fresh veggies, chia seed sprouts, and two tasty spreads assembled on multigrain bread.

6 slices **multigrain bread or other bread**

½ cup **Cha-Cha Chia Seed Dressing** (page 30)

½ cup **hummus**

2 large leaves **leaf lettuce or other lettuce**

4 slices **tomato**

½ **Hass avocado, pitted and thinly sliced**

¼ **red onion, thinly sliced**

½ cup shredded **carrots**

¼ cup thinly sliced **radishes**

⅔ cup **Chia Seed Sprouts** (page 28)

Lightly toast the bread slices. Put the toasted bread slices on a large cutting board or work surface. Spread 2 tablespoons of the dressing on 4 of the slices. Spread 2 tablespoons of the hummus on both sides of the remaining 2 slices.

To assemble the sandwiches, on top of 2 of the dressing-covered bread slices, put 1 lettuce leaf, 2 slices of tomato, half of the avocado, and half of the onion. Top with the 2 hummus-covered bread slices. On each of those bread slices, arrange half of the carrots, half of the radishes, and half of the sprouts. Put the remaining 2 dressing-covered bread slices (dressing-side down) on top of the vegetables and gently press down on each sandwich.

Secure the layered sandwiches with toothpicks and carefully slice each sandwich in half diagonally. Serve the sandwiches immediately, wrap them tightly in waxed paper or plastic wrap, or put them in an airtight container. Stored in the refrigerator, California Club Sandwiches will keep for 1 to 2 days.

VARIATIONS: Replace the Cha-Cha Chia Seed Dressing or hummus with vegan mayonnaise, spicy brown or Dijon mustard, or another spread of choice. For the lettuce leaves, you can substitute other varieties of leafy greens, such as arugula or spinach. If you like, include slices of vegan cheese, baked tofu, tempeh bacon, or meatless deli-style slices when you assemble the sandwiches.

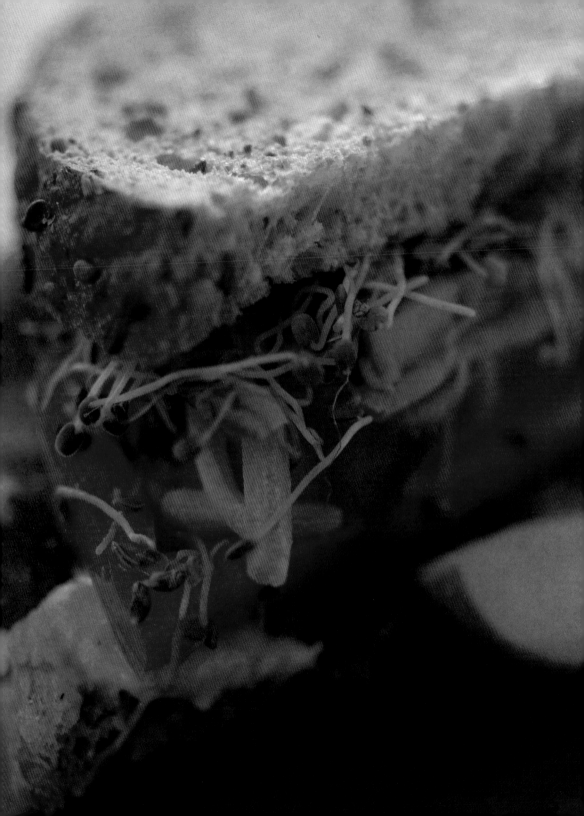

creamy Roasted Tomato Soup

YIELD: 8 CUPS, 8 SERVINGS

Aromatic vegetables, chili powder, smoked paprika, and fire-roasted tomatoes deepen the flavor of this classic tomato soup. A quick sunflower and chia seed cream adds a slight thickness and richness.

SOUP

¾ cup diced **yellow onion**

1 large stalk **celery, diced**

1½ teaspoons **olive oil**

1 tablespoon **minced garlic**

1 (28-ounce) can **fire-roasted crushed tomatoes**

3 cups no-salt-added **vegetable broth or water**

2 tablespoons no-salt-added **tomato paste**

1 **bay leaf**

1 teaspoon **chili powder**

1 teaspoon **smoked paprika**

¾ teaspoon **sea salt**

¼ teaspoon **freshly ground pepper**

To make the soup, put the onion, celery, and olive oil in a large pot and cook over medium heat, stirring occasionally, for 3 minutes to soften. Add the garlic and cook, stirring occasionally, for 1 minute.

Add the crushed tomatoes, vegetable broth, tomato paste, bay leaf, chili powder, smoked paprika, salt, and pepper and stir until well combined. Bring to a boil over high heat. Cover, decrease the heat to low, and simmer for 30 minutes.

SUNFLOWER AND CHIA SEED CREAM

½ cup **raw or roasted sunflower seeds**

2 tablespoons **chia seeds**

1 cup **water**

1 tablespoon **nutritional yeast flakes**

While the soup is simmering, make the Sunflower and Chia Seed Cream. Put the sunflower seeds and chia seeds in a blender and process until finely ground. Add the water and nutritional yeast flakes and process until smooth. Let sit in the blender for 10 minutes to thicken.

Remove the soup from the heat. Add half of the soup to the blender with the Sunflower and Chia Seed Cream and process until completely smooth, stopping occasionally to scrape down the sides of the blender jar with a rubber spatula. Transfer to a large bowl. Process the remaining half of the soup until smooth. Return all of the blended soup to the large pot and stir until well combined. Serve hot.

VARIATIONS: For a slightly chunky soup, only process two-thirds of the soup mixture. For a spicy soup, add ½ teaspoon of chipotle chili powder or cayenne. For a milder soup, use a 28-ounce can of plain no-salt-added crushed tomatoes, omit the chili powder, and replace the smoked paprika with standard sweet paprika.

supper selections

Au Gratin Vegetable *casserole*

YIELD: 9 CUPS, 9 SERVINGS

Nondairy milk, nutritional yeast flakes, chia seeds, and savory seasonings make a cheesy-tasting sauce that covers alternating layers of potatoes and vegetables. A breadcrumb topping helps transform the mixture into a baked casserole that's sure to satisfy any comfort-food cravings.

3 cups **nondairy milk**

⅔ cup **nutritional yeast flakes**

1½ tablespoons **chia seeds**

1½ tablespoons **garlic powder**

1½ tablespoons **onion powder**

1 teaspoon **paprika or smoked paprika**

½ teaspoon **dry mustard**

½ teaspoon **sea salt or seasoned salt**

½ teaspoon **freshly ground pepper**

2 pounds **red-skinned potatoes, scrubbed and thinly sliced**

1 (16-ounce) package **frozen California vegetable blend (broccoli, cauliflower, and carrots)**

½ cup **fresh or dry breadcrumbs**

Preheat the oven to 375 degrees F. Lightly oil a 13 x 9-inch baking pan or mist it with cooking spray.

Put the nondairy milk, nutritional yeast flakes, chia seeds, garlic powder, onion powder, paprika, dry mustard, salt, and pepper in small bowl and whisk until well combined.

Layer half of the potato slices in the prepared baking pan. Top with the vegetable blend, 1 cup of the nondairy milk mixture, and then the remaining potato slices. Pour the remaining nondairy milk mixture over the top and shake the pan gently to allow some of the liquid to sink into the layered ingredients. Evenly sprinkle the breadcrumbs over the top.

Bake for 45 to 50 minutes, or until the potatoes are fork-tender. Let cool for 5 minutes before serving.

VARIATIONS: Replace the red-skinned potatoes with Yukon gold potatoes, or replace all of the potatoes with 2 pounds of turnips or rutabagas, peeled and thinly sliced.

seed-crusted Tofu Cutlets

YIELD: 8 PIECES, 4 SERVINGS

Slices of tofu are first bathed in a tangy marinade and then coated in a three-seed blend. Instead of being fried, these tofu cutlets are baked to perfection.

1 pound **firm or extra-firm tofu**

2 tablespoons **reduced-sodium soy sauce**

1½ tablespoons **nutritional yeast flakes**

1 tablespoon **minced garlic**

1 tablespoon **balsamic vinegar**

1 tablespoon **maple syrup or agave nectar**

1 tablespoon **spicy brown mustard or Dijon mustard**

1 tablespoon **toasted sesame oil**

5 tablespoons **raw sesame seeds**

5 tablespoons **hempseeds**

2½ tablespoons **chia seeds**

Squeeze the block of tofu over the sink to remove any excess water. Put the tofu in a colander in the sink, cover with a plate, and put a 28-ounce can on top of the plate. Let the tofu press for 20 minutes.

Cut the pressed tofu lengthwise into 8 slices. Put the slices in a single layer in an 11 x 7-inch baking pan. Using a fork, pierce each slice of tofu several times along its length. Flip the slices over and pierce the other side.

Put the soy sauce, ½ tablespoon of the nutritional yeast flakes, garlic, vinegar, maple syrup, mustard, and sesame oil in a small bowl and stir until well combined. Pour the mixture over the tofu and flip each slice to evenly coat all sides. Put the baking pan in the refrigerator and let the tofu marinate for 1 to 4 hours.

Preheat the oven to 425 degrees F. Line a baking sheet with parchment paper or a silicone baking mat.

Put the remaining tablespoon of nutritional yeast flakes and the sesame seeds, hempseeds, and chia seeds on plate. Stir until well combined.

To coat the tofu, work with 1 piece at a time. Put each piece into the seed mixture, pressing down slightly and flipping it over as needed until evenly coated on all sides. Transfer to the prepared baking sheet. Bake for 20 minutes.

Remove the baking sheet from the oven. Flip over the cutlets with a spatula. Bake for 15 to 20 minutes longer, until the seeds are fragrant and the cutlets are golden brown. Serve hot or cold.

SEED-CRUSTED TEMPEH CUTLETS: Replace the block of tofu with 2 (8-ounce) packages of tempeh. Cut each package of tempeh into 4 pieces and proceed as directed.

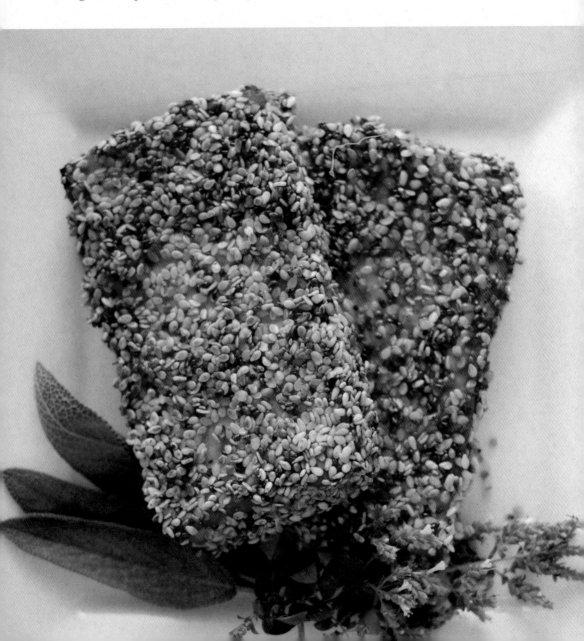

Chia Seed and Veggie *stir-fry*

YIELD: 6 CUPS, 6 SERVINGS

In a slight departure from convention, here a colorful blend of fresh veggies is quickly stir-fried and then covered in a sweet-and-sour sauce thickened with chia seeds rather than the typical cornstarch. Serve this stir-fry as a main dish atop cooked rice, grains, or noodles, or as a side dish as part of an Asian-style meal.

CHIA-THICKENED STIR-FRY SAUCE

¼ cup **reduced-sodium soy sauce**

2 tablespoons **brown rice vinegar**

2 tablespoons **ketchup**

1½ tablespoons **peeled and grated fresh ginger**

1½ tablespoons **minced garlic**

1 tablespoon **agave nectar**

1 tablespoon **chia seeds**

1 tablespoon **toasted sesame oil**

¼ teaspoon **dry mustard**

¼ teaspoon **crushed red pepper flakes**

¼ teaspoon **freshly ground pepper**

To make the sauce, put the soy sauce, vinegar, ketchup, ginger, garlic, agave nectar, chia seeds, sesame oil, dry mustard, red pepper flakes, and pepper in a small bowl. Whisk until well combined. Let thicken for 5 minutes.

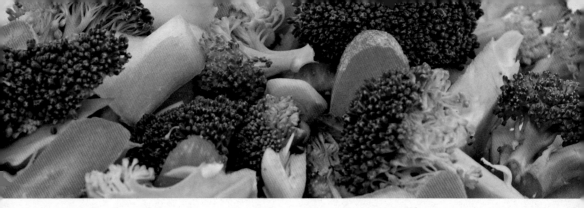

STIR-FRY

2 cups small **broccoli florets**

1 small **red or yellow onion,** cut into half-moons

2 large **carrots,** thinly sliced diagonally

½ **red bell pepper,** quartered lengthwise and thinly sliced

1½ teaspoons **toasted sesame oil**

1 cup shredded **green cabbage** or Savoy cabbage

1 cup shredded **red cabbage**

⅓ cup chopped **fresh cilantro**

¼ cup thinly sliced **green onion**

1½ teaspoons **chia seeds**

1½ teaspoons **raw or roasted sesame seeds**

Sea salt

Freshly ground pepper

To make the stir-fry, put the broccoli, red onion, carrots, bell pepper, and sesame oil in a large nonstick skillet or wok and cook over medium-high heat, stirring occasionally, for 5 minutes. Add the green cabbage and red cabbage and cook, stirring occasionally, until the vegetables are crisp-tender, 1 to 2 minutes.

Add the sauce, cilantro, green onion, chia seeds, and sesame seeds and stir until well combined. Season with salt and pepper to taste. Serve immediately.

TIP: Add or substitute other fresh or frozen vegetables to suit your taste.

VARIATION: Add 1 cup of finely cubed seitan, tofu, or tempeh to the stir-frying vegetables.

Cashew and Veggie *à la king*

YIELD: 4 CUPS, 4 SERVINGS

A tasty blend of sautéed veggies and chickpeas bathed in a cashew gravy thickened with chia seeds makes for a winning combination. Serve this revamped and animal-free version of chicken à la king over rice, whole grains, noodles, toast points, or split biscuits.

CASHEW AND CHIA SEED GRAVY

⅓ cup **raw cashews**

1½ tablespoons **chia seeds**

2½ cups **water**

2½ tablespoons **nutritional yeast flakes**

2½ tablespoons **reduced-sodium soy sauce**

1 tablespoon **onion powder**

1 tablespoon **garlic powder**

½ teaspoon **poultry seasoning blend,** or ¼ teaspoon dried thyme and ¼ teaspoon ground sage

⅛ teaspoon **freshly ground pepper**

To make the gravy, put the cashews and chia seeds in a blender and process until finely ground. Scrape down the sides of the blender jar with a rubber spatula. Add 1 cup of the water and process until smooth. Scrape down the sides of the blender jar with a rubber spatula. Add the remaining 1½ cups of water and the nutritional yeast flakes, soy sauce, onion powder, garlic powder, poultry seasoning, and pepper and process until well combined.

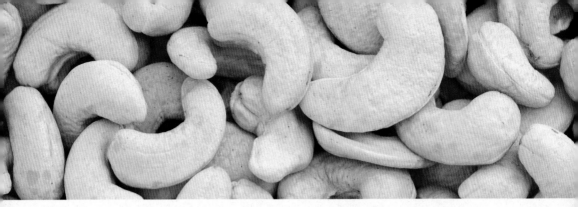

VEGGIE BLEND

¾ cup diced **yellow onion**

¾ cup diced **carrot**

½ cup diced **celery**

½ cup diced **green bell pepper**

½ cup diced **red bell pepper**

1½ teaspoons **olive oil or other oil**

1 (15-ounce) can **chickpeas**, drained and rinsed

½ cup **fresh or frozen peas**

¼ cup chopped **fresh parsley**, lightly packed

Sea salt

Freshly ground pepper

To make the veggie blend, put the onion, carrot, celery, green bell pepper, red bell pepper, and oil in a large saucepan and cook over medium heat, stirring occasionally, until the vegetables are soft, 7 to 10 minutes.

Add the gravy and cook, stirring occasionally, until thickened, 3 to 5 minutes. Add the chickpeas, peas, and parsley and stir until well combined. Season with salt and pepper to taste. Serve hot.

TIP: For an even heartier dish, add ¾ cup of finely cubed seitan, tofu, or tempeh to the veggie blend as it cooks.

loaded Bean Burritos with Chia Seed Salsa

Prevent freshly made salsa from being too watery simply by adding some chia seeds. This technique can help to keep rolled burritos from getting soggy, or if you're eating a burrito on the go, to avoid excess juices running down your chin.

CHIA SEED SALSA (3½ CUPS)

2 cups diced **tomatoes**

½ cup diced **green bell pepper**

½ cup diced **red or orange bell pepper**

½ cup diced **red or yellow onion**

⅓ cup chopped **fresh cilantro**, lightly packed

¼ cup thinly sliced **green onion**

½ **jalapeño chile**, seeded and finely diced

Juice of 1 **lime** (about 2 tablespoons)

1 tablespoon **minced garlic**

2 teaspoons **chia seeds**

1 teaspoon **sea salt**

½ teaspoon **freshly ground pepper**

½ teaspoon **smoked paprika**

To make the salsa, put the tomatoes, green bell pepper, red bell pepper, red onion, cilantro, green onion, chile, lime juice, garlic, chia seeds, salt, pepper, and smoked paprika in a large bowl and stir until well combined. Let sit for 15 minutes to allow the flavors to blend and the chia seeds to slightly thicken the salsa.

For easier rolling, warm each tortilla in a large skillet over medium heat for 1 to 2 minutes per side. Alternatively, warm each tortilla in the microwave for 20 to 30 seconds.

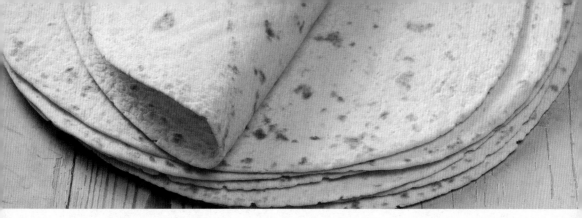

BURRITOS

4 (8-inch) **flour tortillas or gluten-free tortillas**

1 (15-ounce) can **reduced-sodium vegetarian refried beans,** warmed

½ cup shredded **vegan cheese**

1 Hass **avocado,** diced

¼ cup **vegan sour cream**

1 cup shredded **lettuce**

To assemble each burrito, put 1 tortilla flat on a large cutting board or work surface. Spread ⅓ cup of the refried beans in a horizontal line in the center of the tortilla. On top, layer in order, 2 tablespoons of the vegan cheese, one-quarter of the avocado, 1 tablespoon of the vegan sour cream, ¼ cup of the Chia Seed Salsa, and ¼ cup of the lettuce. (Store leftover salsa in a covered container in the refrigerator to use with other dishes.)

To roll each burrito, fold the bottom half of the tortilla over the filling, fold in each side toward the center over the filling, and roll up from the bottom edge to enclose the filling. Put the burrito seam-side down on a plate. Repeat the assembly and rolling procedure with the remaining tortillas and filling ingredients. Serve immediately.

INSIDE-OUT BURRITOS: Omit the lettuce and vegan sour cream in the assembly procedure of each burrito. For each serving, put the shredded lettuce in the center of the plate, and put the rolled burrito seam-side down on top of the lettuce. Garnish each burrito with an additional ⅓ cup of Chia Seed Salsa and 1 tablespoon of the vegan sour cream.

Azteca *quinoa*

Some of the earliest crops cultivated by the indigenous people of Central and South America included corn, beans, squash, quinoa, and chia seeds. These key ingredients combine in this recipe to create a flavorful and filling option that works as either a main dish or a side dish.

2 cups **water**

1 cup **quinoa**, well rinsed

1½ cups seeded and cubed **delicata squash** or other winter squash (about half a squash)

1 tablespoon **olive oil**

½ cup diced **red onion**

½ cup diced **red bell pepper**

⅔ cup **fresh or frozen corn kernels**

1 tablespoon **minced garlic**

1 teaspoon **chili powder**

1 teaspoon **ground cumin**

1 teaspoon **sea salt**

½ teaspoon **freshly ground pepper**

⅛ teaspoon **cayenne or chipotle chili powder**

¾ cup cooked or canned **kidney, red, or black beans,** drained and rinsed

¼ cup **raw or roasted pumpkin seeds**

¼ cup chopped **fresh cilantro or parsley,** lightly packed

2 tablespoons **chia seeds**

1 tablespoon **nutritional yeast flakes**

Put the water and quinoa in a medium saucepan and bring to a boil over high heat. Cover, decrease the heat to low, and cook until the quinoa is tender and all of the water is absorbed, 15 to 18 minutes. Remove from the heat.

While the quinoa is cooking, put the squash and oil in a large cast-iron or non-stick skillet and cook over medium heat, stirring occasionally, for 7 minutes. Add the onion and bell pepper and cook, stirring occasionally, for 5 minutes.

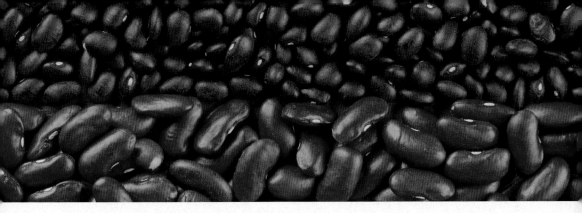

Add the corn, garlic, chili powder, cumin, salt, pepper, and cayenne and cook, stirring occasionally, until the squash is tender, 2 to 3 minutes. Remove from the heat.

Fluff the quinoa with a fork to separate the grains. Add the quinoa, beans, pumpkin seeds, cilantro, chia seeds, and nutritional yeast flakes to the squash mixture and stir until well combined. Serve hot, cold, or at room temperature.

TIPS: For increased nutrition and eye appeal, use a tricolor quinoa blend. For a heartier dish, put individual servings on a bed of lettuce or mixed greens.

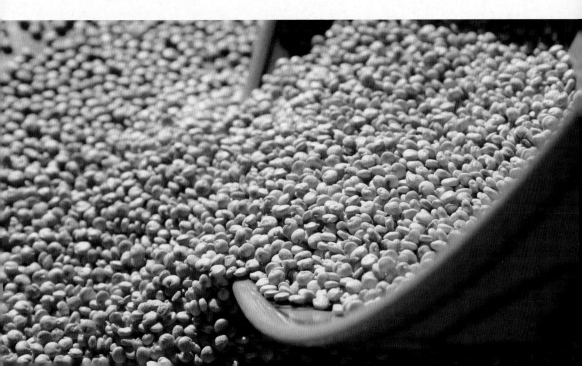

sweets and treats

Raw Energy *snacks*

Rather than reaching for a protein bar when you're in need of an energy boost after working out, have one or two of these tasty treats instead. They're made with several nutritious ingredients hailed as superfoods, including maca powder, cacao nibs, goji berries, hempseeds, and, of course, chia.

⅓ cup **dried cranberries**

⅓ cup **raisins**

¼ cup **goji berries**

¼ cup **cacao nibs**

¼ cup **hempseeds**

¼ cup **raw pumpkin seeds**

¼ cup **raw sunflower seeds**

¼ cup **unsweetened shredded dried coconut**

1 tablespoon **maca powder**

¾ teaspoon **ground cinnamon**

3½ tablespoons **Chia Seed Gel** (page 16)

Put the cranberries, raisins, goji berries, cacao nibs, hempseeds, pumpkin seeds, sunflower seeds, coconut, maca powder, and cinnamon in a food processor and process just until slightly chunky. Add the Chia Seed Gel and process briefly, just until well combined. Transfer the mixture to a small bowl and refrigerate for 1 hour.

To form the mixture, dampen your hands with water. Form the mixture into 12 (1½-inch) balls. Serve immediately if desired. Stored in an airtight container in the refrigerator, Raw Energy Snacks will keep for 7 days.

53

multigrain and Fruit Jam Bars

YIELD: 12 BARS

Soft and sweet, these bars blend rolled oats, barley flour, coconut, nuts, and seeds with a middle layer of homemade fruit jam. Enjoy these wholesome snacks on the go or after school or work.

CHIA-ENHANCED FRUIT JAM

1 cup **fresh berries or chopped fruit or frozen berries or fruit, thawed**

1 tablespoon **agave nectar or other sweetener**

½ teaspoon **vanilla extract**

2 teaspoons **chia seeds**

To make the jam, put the berries, agave nectar, and vanilla extract in a food processor and process just until slightly chunky. Scrape down the sides of the container with a rubber spatula. Add the chia seeds and process for 30 seconds. Let the mixture sit for 10 minutes. Process the jam for 10 seconds to break up any clumps of chia seeds. Let sit for 5 to 10 minutes longer until thickened.

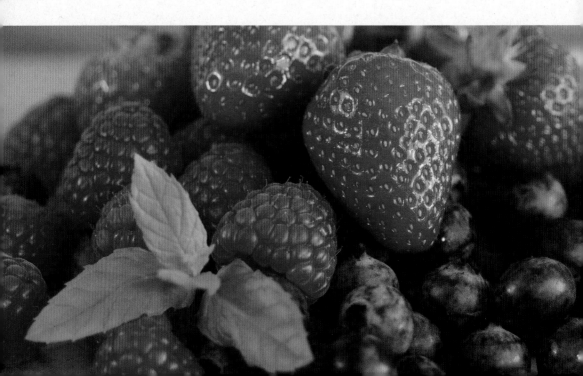

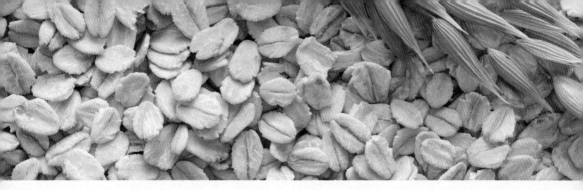

MULTIGRAIN BASE

1½ cups **old-fashioned rolled oats**

1 cup **barley flour or other flour**

½ cup **light or dark brown sugar,** lightly packed

1½ teaspoons **ground cinnamon**

¾ teaspoon aluminum-free **baking powder**

¼ teaspoon **sea salt**

½ cup melted **coconut oil or nonhydrogenated vegan margarine,** melted

⅓ cup **water**

1½ teaspoons **vanilla extract**

⅓ cup coarsely chopped **raw walnuts or almonds**

¼ cup **raw sunflower seeds**

3 tablespoons **unsweetened shredded dried coconut**

2 tablespoons **chia seeds**

To make the multigrain base, preheat the oven to 375 degrees F. Line an 8-inch square baking pan with parchment paper, allowing the paper to slightly drape over two opposite sides of the pan.

Put the oats, barley flour, brown sugar, cinnamon, baking powder, and salt in a large bowl and stir until well combined. Add the coconut oil, water, and vanilla extract and use your fingers to work them into the dry ingredients. Add the walnuts, sunflower seeds, coconut, and chia seeds and stir until well combined.

Transfer half of the oat mixture to the prepared pan. Using your fingers, firmly press the oat mixture into an even layer. Evenly spread the jam over the oat mixture. Sprinkle the remaining half of the oat mixture over the jam, using your fingers to gently press it into an even layer.

Bake for 30 to 35 minutes, until golden brown. Let cool completely in the pan. Run a knife around the edges of the pan, and then use the parchment paper to lift the bars out of the pan. Cut into 12 squares. Stored in an airtight container at room temperature, Multigrain and Fruit Jam Bars will keep for 3 to 5 days.

almond butter–Chocolate Chip Cookies

YIELD: 24 COOKIES

Coconut oil, two types of sugar, and almond butter nicely complement each other and also impart a slightly caramel flavor to these chewy cookies. They are studded with chocolate chips, almonds, and coconut.

⅔ cup **light or dark brown sugar,** lightly packed

⅓ cup melted **coconut oil**

⅓ cup **almond butter**

⅓ cup **unbleached cane sugar**

¼ cup **Chia Seed Gel** (page 16)

¼ cup **water**

1½ teaspoons **vanilla extract**

2¼ cups **whole wheat pastry flour**

¾ teaspoon **aluminum-free baking powder**

¾ teaspoon **baking soda**

½ teaspoon **sea salt**

¾ cup vegan **chocolate chips**

⅓ cup coarsely chopped **almonds**

3 tablespoons **unsweetened shredded dried coconut**

Preheat the oven to 375 degrees F. Line two large baking sheets with parchment paper or silicone baking mats.

Put the brown sugar, coconut oil, almond butter, unbleached sugar, Chia Seed Gel, water, and vanilla extract in a large bowl and whisk until well combined. Put the flour, baking powder, baking soda, and salt in a medium bowl and stir until well combined. Add the dry ingredients to the wet ingredients and stir until well combined. Using your hands, work in the chocolate chips, almonds, and coconut.

Drop the dough on the prepared baking sheets, using a 1½-inch scoop or a heaping tablespoonful for each cookie, spacing them about 2 inches apart. Flatten each cookie slightly with your fingertips.

Bake one sheet at a time, 13 minutes for soft cookies or 15 minutes for crunchy cookies. The cookies should be golden brown on the bottom and around the edges. Let the cookies cool on the baking sheet for 2 minutes before transferring them to a rack to cool completely. Stored in an airtight container at room temperature, Almond Butter–Chocolate Chip Cookies will keep for 5 to 7 days.

VARIATIONS: Replace the almond butter with another variety of nut or seed butter (such as cashew, sunflower, or peanut) and the chopped almonds with other nuts (such as cashews, pecans, or walnuts).

WHEAT-FREE ALMOND BUTTER–CHOCOLATE CHIP COOKIES: Replace the whole wheat pastry flour with spelt flour or barley flour.

GLUTEN-FREE ALMOND BUTTER–CHOCOLATE CHIP COOKIES: Replace the whole wheat pastry flour with a gluten-free baking mix and add 1½ teaspoons of xanthan gum.

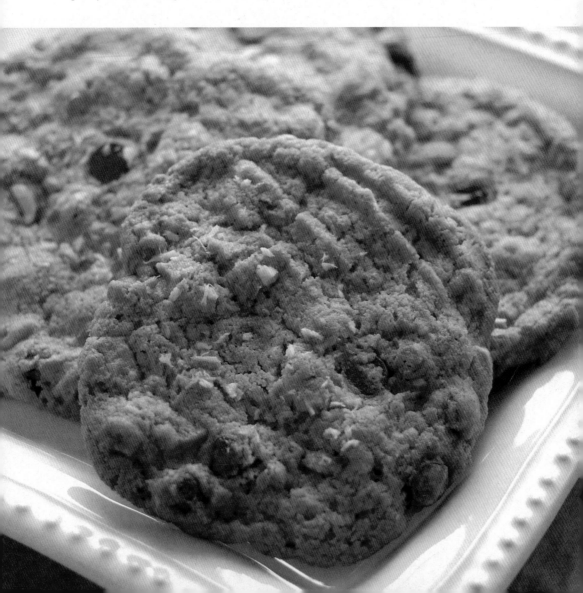

chocolate **Chia Pudding**

YIELD: 2 CUPS, 4 SERVINGS

This no-cook pudding is so simple to make, yet it tastes amazingly rich and creamy. It's sure to become your go-to guilt-free treat for satisfying your chocolate cravings.

2 cups **chocolate nondairy milk,** such as almond milk, soy milk, or coconut milk beverage

2 tablespoons **agave nectar**

½ teaspoon **vanilla extract**

⅓ cup **chia seeds**

Topping options: cacao nibs, coarsely chopped nuts, unsweetened shredded dried coconut, sliced strawberries, or red raspberries

Put the nondairy milk, agave nectar, and vanilla extract in a medium bowl and whisk until well combined. Add the chia seeds and whisk until well combined. Let thicken for 10 minutes. Whisk the mixture again to break up any clumps of chia seeds.

Put the mixture in the refrigerator until the chia seeds swell and thicken the mixture to a pudding-like consistency, about 1 hour.

Evenly divide the pudding among four bowls. Serve immediately or refrigerate. Garnish with one or more of the topping options as desired.

CHOCOLATE-MINT OR CAROB CHIA PUDDING: Replace the chocolate nondairy milk with chocolate-mint or carob nondairy milk.

VANILLA CHIA PUDDING: Replace the chocolate nondairy milk with vanilla nondairy milk and add an additional ½ teaspoon of vanilla extract.

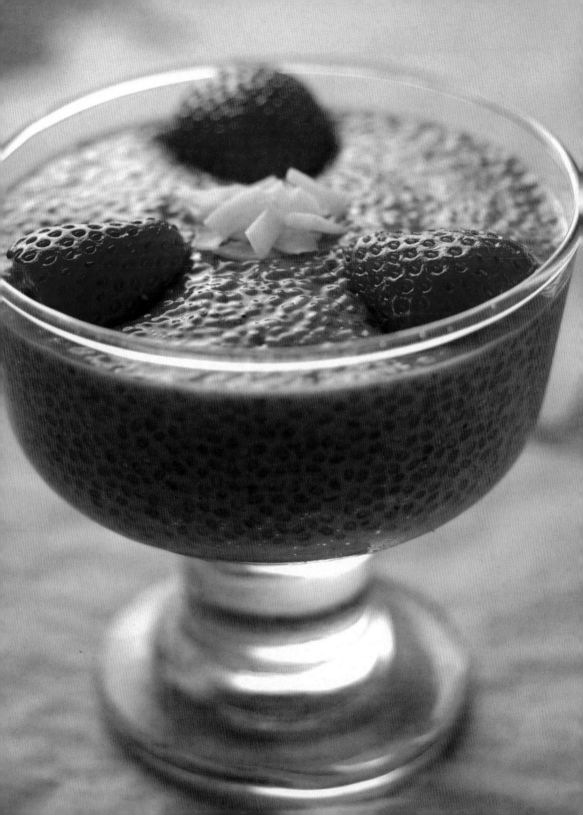

lemon-berry **Cake**

Using both the zest and juice of a fresh lemon heightens the flavor of the sweet and juicy berries. Instead of the large amounts of oil found in most baked goods, yogurt gives this low-fat cake a moist, tender crumb. Serve it plain, with a light dusting of powdered sugar, or topped with a scoop of sorbet or nondairy ice cream and additional berries.

1¾ cups **unbleached flour or whole wheat pastry flour**

¾ cup **unbleached cane sugar**

1 teaspoon **baking soda**

¼ teaspoon **aluminum-free baking powder**

¼ teaspoon **sea salt**

½ cup **water**

⅓ cup **vanilla or lemon vegan yogurt**

Zest and juice of 1 **lemon** (1½ teaspoons zest and ¼ cup juice)

2 tablespoons **Chia Seed Gel** (page 16)

1 tablespoon **safflower oil or other oil**

1 teaspoon **vanilla extract**

½ cup **fresh or frozen berries,** such as blueberries, blackberries, or red raspberries

Preheat the oven to 350 degrees F. Lightly oil an 8-inch round or square baking pan or mist it with cooking spray.

Put the flour, sugar, baking soda, baking powder, and salt in a large bowl and whisk until well combined. Put the water, vegan yogurt, lemon zest and juice, Chia Seed Gel, oil, and vanilla extract in a small bowl and whisk until well combined. Add the wet ingredients to the dry ingredients and whisk until completely smooth. Gently stir in the berries.

Scrape the batter into the prepared pan. Bake for 30 to 35 minutes, or until a toothpick inserted in the center comes out clean. Serve warm or at room temperature. Stored at room temperature in an airtight container or covered with plastic wrap, Lemon-Berry Cake will keep for 3 to 5 days.

WHEAT-FREE LEMON-BERRY CAKE: Replace the unbleached flour with spelt flour.

GLUTEN-FREE LEMON-BERRY CAKE: Replace the unbleached flour with a gluten-free baking mix and add ½ teaspoon xanthan gum.

ORANGE-CRANBERRY CAKE: Replace the lemon zest and juice with the zest of 1 orange and ¼ cup of orange juice, and use ⅔ cup of fresh or frozen cranberries for the berries.

Fruit-and-Cream *chia pops*

YIELD: 4 POPS

Much healthier than store-bought pops, these homemade frozen treats blend sweet and juicy fruit or berries with coconut milk beverage. Stock the freezer with these refreshing pops for an impromptu summer snack.

½ cup **vanilla coconut milk beverage**

2 tablespoons **agave nectar or brown rice syrup**

2 tablespoons **chia seeds**

¾ cup coarsely chopped **fruit** (such as banana, mango, or peach) or berries (such as blueberries, red raspberries, or strawberries)

Put the coconut milk beverage, agave nectar, and chia seeds in a blender or food processor and process for 30 seconds. Let thicken for 5 minutes. Scrape down the sides of the container with a rubber spatula. Add the fruit and pulse several times to combine. Alternatively, for a smoother texture, process all of the ingredients until smooth.

Pour the mixture into 4 (3-ounce) ice-pop molds, dividing it evenly. Insert the mold sticks and freeze until frozen solid, 8 to 12 hours.

For easy removal from the molds, let the frozen pops sit at room temperature for 3 to 4 minutes or dip the molds quickly in hot water. Serve immediately. Stored in their molds in the freezer, Fruit-and-Cream Chia Pops will keep for 1 month.

VARIATION: Substitute other varieties of fresh fruit or berries depending on seasonal availability or your preference, or use frozen fruits if desired.

SMOOTHIE POPS: Blend 2 tablespoons of chia seeds with 1 cup of leftover smoothie. Pour into ice-pop molds and freeze.

ABOUT THE AUTHOR

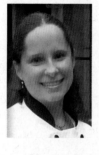

Beverly Lynn Bennett is an experienced vegan chef and baker, writer, and animal advocate who is passionate about showing the world how easy, delicious, and healthy it is to live and eat as a vegan. A certified food-service operations manager, she earned her culinary arts degree in 1988 from the University of Akron, Ohio, and in the following years worked in and managed vegan and vegetarian restaurants and natural food stores.

Vegan since the early 1990s, Beverly is the author of *Vegan Bites: Recipes for Singles* and *The Complete Idiot's Guide to Vegan Slow Cooking.* She is also the coauthor of *The Complete Idiot's Guide to Vegan Living, The Complete Idiot's Guide to Vegan Cooking,* and *The Complete Idiot's Guide to Gluten-Free Vegan Cooking.* Her work has appeared in many national and international print publications, on public television and DVD, and all over the web. She has hosted the popular Vegan Chef website at VeganChef.com since 1999 and has been a regular columnist for *VegNews* magazine since 2002.

Beverly currently lives and works in Eugene, Oregon, where her love of organic, healthy, and vibrant foods fuels a passion for developing innovative vegan recipes. When she isn't hard at work in the kitchen, she can often be found frequenting farmers' markets and educating others on issues relating to veganism and health through cooking demos and speaking engagements.

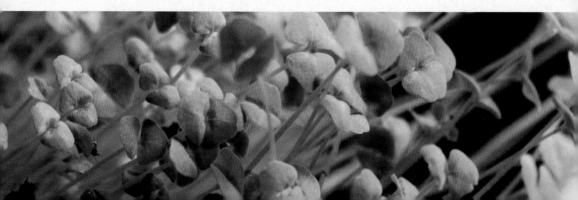

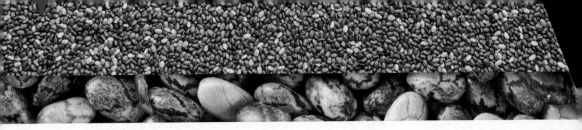

© 2014 Beverly Lynn Bennett

Food photography: Andrew Schmidt, 123 RF
Food styling: Ron Maxen
Book design, photo editing: John Wincek
Editing: Beth Geisler, Jo Stepaniak

Pictured on front cover: Seed-Crusted Tofu Cutlets, page 42

Published by **Books Alive**
PO Box 99
Summertown, TN 38483
931-964-3571
888-260-8458
www.bookpubco.com

ISBN: 978-1-155312-049-0

Printed in Hong Kong

Library of Congress Cataloging-in-Publication Data

Bennett, Beverly Lynn.
  Chia : using the ancient superfood / Beverly Lynn Bennett.
    pages cm
  Includes bibliographical references and index.
  ISBN 978-1-55312-049-0 (pbk.) — ISBN 978-1-55312-097-1 (e-book)
1. Chia. 2. Natural foods I. Title.
  TX558.C38.B46 2014
  641.3'02—dc23

                   2013035125

Note: The recipes in this book are by no means to be taken as therapeutic. They simply promote the philosophy of both the authors and Books Alive in relation to whole foods, health, and nutrition, while incorporating the practical advice given by the authors in the first section of the book.

It is your constitutional right to educate yourself in health and medical knowledge, to seek helpful information, and to make use of it for your own benefit and for that of your family. You are the one responsible for your health. In order to make decisions in all health matters, you must educate yourself. With this book and the guidance of a naturopath or alternative medical doctor, you will learn what is needed to achieve optimal health.

Those individuals currently taking pharmaceutical prescription drugs will want to talk to their healthcare professionals about the negative effects that the drugs can have on herbal remedies and nutritional supplements, before combining them.

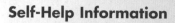
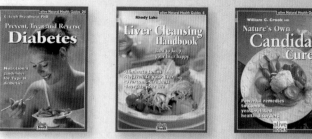
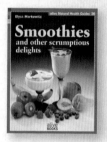
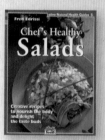
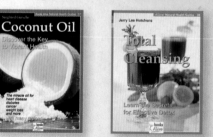
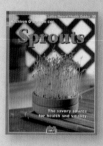
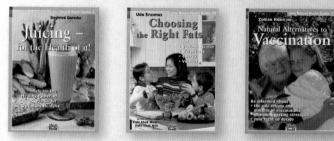

ALIVE NATURAL HEALTH GUIDES